THE HONEY POWER

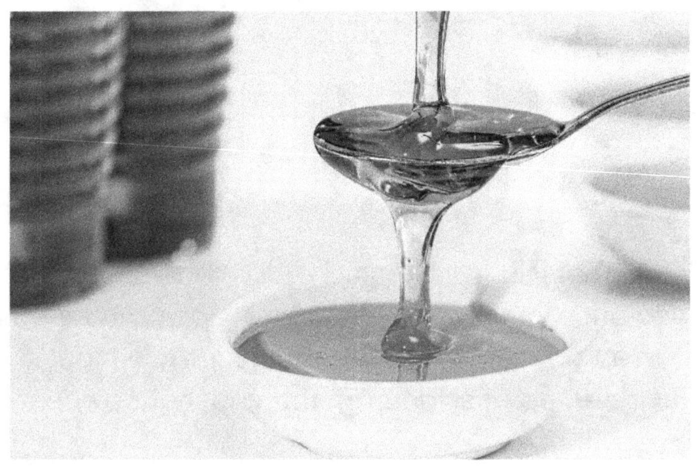

Discovering The Health Benefits Of Sweetner And The Natural Remedies

Shane Ramiro

Table of contents

Introduction

In a quaint village nestled between rolling hills and meadows, there existed a hidden treasure that bestowed miraculous healing upon its inhabitants. This treasure was none other than the golden elixir produced by the diligent bees – honey. The villagers had long revered the sweet substance not merely for its delectable taste but for its remarkable therapeutic properties.

Legend whispered tales of an ancient beekeeper who discovered the healing powers of honey when his ailing wife experienced a sudden resurgence of health after consuming the nectar regularly. This revelation sparked a profound exploration into the medicinal potential of honey, transcending its role as a mere culinary delight.

As seasons changed, so did the ailments that befell the villagers. From soothing sore throats to accelerating wound healing, honey emerged as a reliable remedy. The locals cultivated a profound respect for the bees, considering them sacred guardians of their well-being.

Word spread beyond the village, drawing curious souls seeking solace from the remarkable healing powers attributed to this golden ambrosia. Scientists and herbalists embarked on journeys to unravel the mysteries of honey's medicinal prowess, conducting studies that confirmed what the villagers had known for generations.

The Healing Powers of Honey became a topic of fascination, a subject of research and admiration worldwide. It wasn't merely a sweetener but a natural healer, a testament to the symbiotic relationship between humans and the tiny, industrious bees. The village, once a hidden sanctuary, now stood as a beacon of health, where the magic of honey transformed lives and ignited a global appreciation for nature's extraordinary remedies.

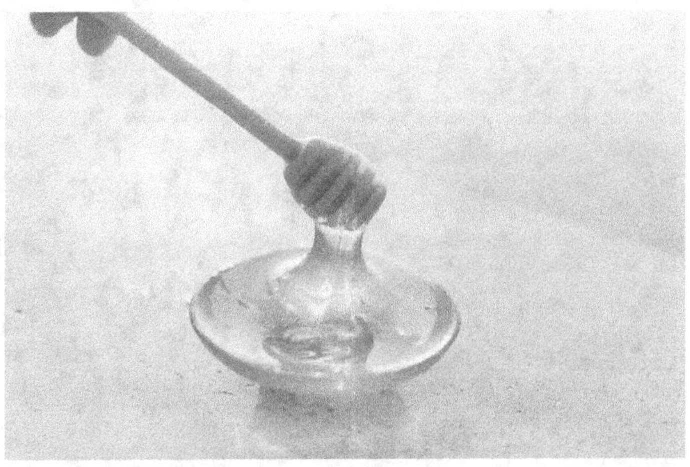

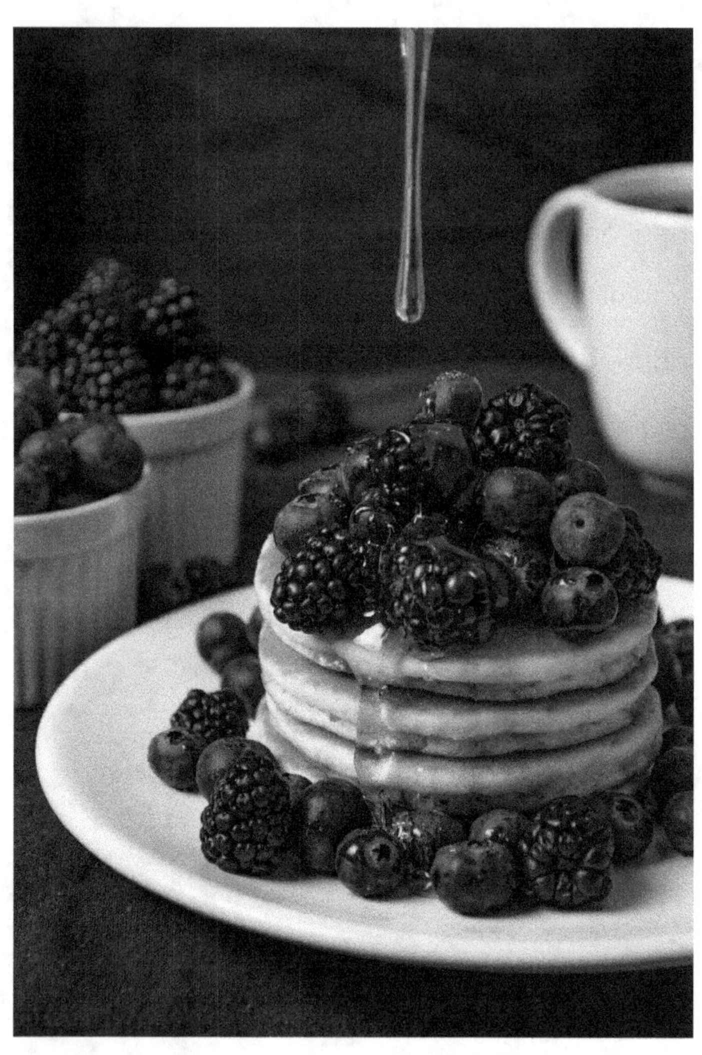

Chapter one

What is Honey

Honey is a natural sweet substance produced by honeybees using nectar from flowers. This complex liquid is composed primarily of sugars such as glucose and fructose, along with water, enzymes, and various other compounds. Bees collect nectar from flowers, transform it within their bodies, and deposit it into honeycombs where the liquid undergoes further processing. The bees then fan the nectar with their wings to reduce its water content, ultimately creating honey.

The color, flavor, and aroma of honey can vary significantly depending on the types of flowers from which the bees collect nectar. This diversity results in a wide range of honey varieties, each with its own distinct characteristics.

Honey has been a staple in human diets for thousands of years, appreciated not only for its sweetness but also for its potential health benefits. Its antimicrobial and antioxidant properties have made it a traditional remedy for various ailments, and it has cultural and historical significance in many societies around the world. In addition to its culinary uses, honey finds applications in skincare, wound healing, and even allergy management.

Overall, honey is a natural and versatile product created by bees, valued for its unique taste and potential health-promoting properties.

Chapter two

The power of Honey

Honey, beyond its exquisite taste and culinary applications, harbors a wealth of remarkable properties that have earned it a revered status throughout history. Its power extends far beyond the realms of a mere sweetener, encompassing a myriad of health, beauty, and therapeutic benefits.

One of the most prominent attributes of honey lies in its potent antimicrobial properties. Rich in natural enzymes and acidic pH, honey creates an inhospitable environment for bacteria and microbes. This has been harnessed for centuries as a topical treatment for wounds and burns, promoting faster healing and minimizing infection risk.

The antioxidants present in honey contribute to its anti-inflammatory effects, making it a soothing remedy for various ailments. From alleviating sore throats with a warm honey and lemon concoction to providing relief for gastrointestinal issues, honey's versatility in addressing internal and external health concerns is unparalleled.

Beyond its medicinal qualities, honey boasts energy-boosting characteristics. Its natural sugars, primarily fructose and glucose, offer a quick and sustained energy release, making it a preferred choice for athletes and those seeking a natural pick-me-up.

The unique composition of honey also renders it an ally in the pursuit of skincare. With its ability to attract and retain moisture, honey is a natural humectant, contributing to skin hydration. Face masks, cleansers, and even wound dressings infused with honey have become popular for their ability to nourish and rejuvenate the skin.

Furthermore, honey has demonstrated potential in managing allergies. Locally sourced honey contains trace amounts of pollen, acting as a natural inoculation against seasonal allergies when consumed regularly.

As science delves deeper into the intricacies of honey, its power continues to unfold, showcasing its potential in diverse fields. From the apothecaries of ancient civilizations to modern research laboratories, honey stands as a testament to nature's ability to provide not only culinary delights but also a myriad of health-enhancing properties. The power of honey, with its ancient origins and modern applications, remains a fascinating testament to the synergy between nature and human well-being.

Chapter three

The Ancient Essential Elixir

Heralded as an ancient essential elixir, honey has transcended epochs, standing as a timeless remedy and culinary treasure. Across the tapestry of civilizations, from the ancient Egyptians to the Greeks and beyond, honey has been revered not merely as a sweet indulgence but as a substance endowed with mystical properties.

In the realm of health, honey's prominence as an elixir traces back to the annals of traditional medicine. Ancient healers recognized its potent antimicrobial and anti-inflammatory attributes, prescribing it for wounds, respiratory ailments, and digestive issues. The elixir's ability to soothe, heal, and fortify the human body earned it a reputation as a life-enriching substance, a sentiment echoed in the writings of historical medical luminaries like Hippocrates.

Culturally, honey assumed a sacred role. In religious ceremonies and rituals, it was offered as a symbol of purity and divine sweetness. The ancient Greeks, attributing its creation to celestial forces, deemed honey the food of the gods—a heavenly elixir connecting mortals to the divine.

As societies traded and interacted along ancient routes, honey became a sought-after commodity, symbolizing prosperity and exotic flavors. Its journey along the Silk Road and other trade routes not only enriched culinary traditions but also fostered cross-cultural exchanges, as honey infused various cuisines with its golden richness.

In the modern era, scientific exploration has unveiled the elixir's intricate composition, revealing a symphony of enzymes, antioxidants, and minerals. Honey's applications have expanded to skincare, where it acts as a natural humectant, preserving moisture and enhancing radiance.

Today, honey endures as an ancient essential elixir, a testament to its enduring appeal and multifaceted virtues. Its golden glow on breakfast tables, in apothecaries, and on skincare shelves resonates with the echoes of centuries, embodying the timeless allure of nature's most enchanting elixir.

Nectar of the gods

Often referred to as the "nectar of the gods," honey has earned this illustrious title through centuries of cultural reverence and appreciation. This evocative phrase captures the essence of honey's divine qualities, celebrating its exquisite taste, natural richness, and the mystical process through which it is created.

In numerous ancient mythologies and religions, honey holds a sacred status. The Greeks believed it to be the food of the gods on Mount Olympus, symbolizing immortality and divine sweetness. In Hinduism, honey is associated with spiritual purity and featured prominently in religious ceremonies.

Beyond its mythological significance, the "nectar of the gods" moniker encapsulates the universal admiration for honey's unrivaled taste. Its distinct flavors, ranging from delicate and floral to robust and earthy, evoke a sensory experience that transcends the ordinary. This divine sweetness has made honey a cherished ingredient in cuisines worldwide, gracing tables with its golden allure.

Moreover, the intricate process of honey creation, orchestrated by the diligent work of bees, adds to its mystical aura. The collaboration between nature and these industrious insects results in a substance that goes beyond a simple sweetener—it becomes a symbol of harmony between the earthly and the ethereal.

Whether drizzled over culinary delights, used in ancient rituals, or praised in poetic verses, honey, as the "nectar of the gods," encapsulates the enchanting blend of flavor, tradition, and natural wonder that has captivated human imagination for millennia.

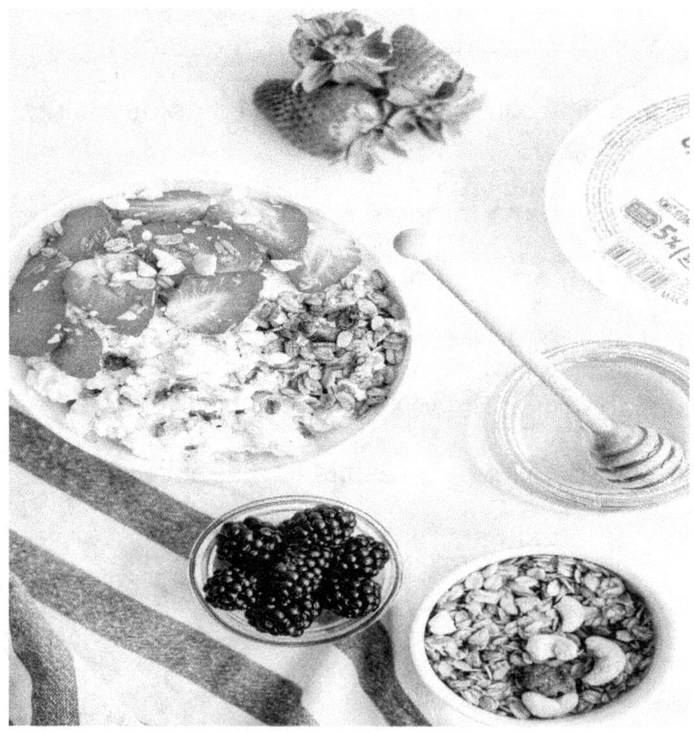

Chapter four

A historical Testimony

In the annals of history, honey emerges as a timeless testimony to the intricate interplay between nature, culture, and human innovation. Archaeological findings indicate that honey was a coveted substance in ancient civilizations, with evidence dating back to the Stone Age. The ancient Egyptians, renowned for their advanced agricultural practices, showcased honey's importance through hieroglyphs depicting beekeeping and honey extraction.

In the Mediterranean, the Greeks and Romans revered honey not only for its sweetness but also for its perceived medicinal properties. Hippocrates, the father of medicine, prescribed honey for various ailments, recognizing its potential to heal wounds and soothe respiratory issues. Across cultures, honey found its place on the tables of royalty, symbolizing wealth and indulgence.

The Silk Road, the ancient trade network connecting the East to the West, played a pivotal role in the spread of honey's allure. As merchants traversed vast landscapes, honey became a coveted commodity, exchanged for its unique flavors and reputed health benefits. This exchange fostered cultural exchanges, with honey leaving an indelible mark on the culinary traditions of diverse societies.

During the Middle Ages, monasteries became centers of beekeeping, with monks tending to beehives and producing honey not only for sustenance but also for medicinal uses. The significance of honey persisted through Renaissance Europe, where it adorned the tables of nobility and was incorporated into the elaborate feasts of the time.

The colonial era witnessed the introduction of European honeybees to the Americas, further intertwining honey with the tapestry of global cultures. As societies evolved, so did the understanding of honey's chemical composition and medicinal properties, leading to its continued use in traditional remedies and modern healthcare practices.

In the 21st century, honey stands as a living historical testament, transcending its ancient roots to find a place in contemporary diets and holistic wellness. From ancient Egyptian tombs to modern supermarket shelves, honey's journey through history reflects the enduring human fascination with this golden elixir—a testimony to its cultural, culinary, and medicinal significance across the ages.

Secret ingredients of honey

The secret ingredients of honey are primarily nectar, collected by bees from flowers, and enzymes produced by the bees. During the honey-making process, bees add their own enzymes to the nectar, transforming it into honey. Additionally, honey contains small amounts of pollen, propolis, and minerals, contributing to its unique flavor and potential health benefits.

Chapter five

The Mediterranean Sweetener

The Mediterranean region is known for its diverse and flavorful honey varieties. The secret to the Mediterranean sweetener lies in the rich nectar from a variety of flowers like thyme, lavender, rosemary, and citrus blossoms. These unique floral sources contribute to the distinct taste and aromatic qualities of Mediterranean honey, making it a sought-after sweetener with a touch of floral complexity.

Honey Flavors

Honey flavors vary widely based on the types of flowers from which bees collect nectar. Some common honey flavors include:

1. **Clover Honey:** Mild and versatile, derived from the nectar of clover blossoms.

2. **Wildflower Honey:** A mix of nectars from various wildflowers, resulting in a nuanced and diverse flavor profile.

3. **Orange Blossom Honey:** Light and citrusy, sourced from orange blossom nectar, providing a delicate and fruity taste.

4. **Lavender Honey:** Infused with the essence of lavender flowers, offering a soothing and aromatic flavor.

5. **Manuka Honey:** Originating from New Zealand, it has a distinct, robust flavor and is renowned for potential health benefits.

6. **Acacia Honey:** Light and mildly sweet, derived from the nectar of acacia blossoms.

7. **Buckwheat Honey:** Dark and rich, with a strong molasses-like flavor, often preferred for its robust taste.

8. **Eucalyptus Honey:** Exhibits a menthol undertone due to bees foraging on eucalyptus blossoms.

The diversity in honey flavors arises from the vast array of flowers bees visit, making honey a complex and delightful natural sweetener.

Healing power varieties

While honey is not a cure-all, some varieties are believed to have potential health benefits due to their unique properties. Here are a few varieties often associated with healing powers:

1. **Manuka Honey:** Known for its antimicrobial properties, especially due to high levels of methylglyoxal (MGO). It is believed to aid in wound healing and have immune-boosting qualities.
2. **Raw Honey:** Unprocessed and unfiltered honey retains more of its natural enzymes and antioxidants, potentially offering anti-inflammatory and antibacterial benefits.
3. **Buckwheat Honey:** With darker color and stronger flavor, it may have higher antioxidant content and is sometimes used to soothe coughs and throat irritation.

4. **Thyme Honey:** Contains compounds
    from thyme flowers, believed to have
    antimicrobial and antioxidant properties.

5. **Eucalyptus Honey:** Known for its
    potential respiratory benefits, it is often
    used to alleviate symptoms of colds and
    respiratory issues.

It's important to note that while these varieties
may have certain beneficial properties,
individual responses can vary, and honey
should not replace professional medical advice
or treatment. Always consult with a healthcare
professional for personalized guidance.

More healing superfoods

While honey itself is considered a natural superfood with potential health benefits, combining it with other nutrient-rich ingredients can enhance its healing properties. Here are some examples:

1. **Turmeric Honey:** Combining honey with anti-inflammatory turmeric may provide a potent blend to support joint health and reduce inflammation.
2. **Ginger Honey:** Ginger's anti-inflammatory and digestive properties, combined with honey, create a soothing blend that may help with digestion and ease nausea.
3. **Cinnamon Honey:** This combination is not only delicious but also thought to

have potential benefits for managing blood sugar levels and providing antioxidants.

4. **Propolis-Infused Honey:** Propolis, a resinous substance collected by bees, is known for its antimicrobial properties. Combining it with honey enhances its immune-boosting potential.

5. **Garlic Honey:** Garlic is well-known for its immune-boosting properties. Combining it with honey can create a flavorful concoction with potential benefits for respiratory health.

Remember, while these combinations may offer additional health benefits, they should not replace a balanced diet, and individual responses can vary.

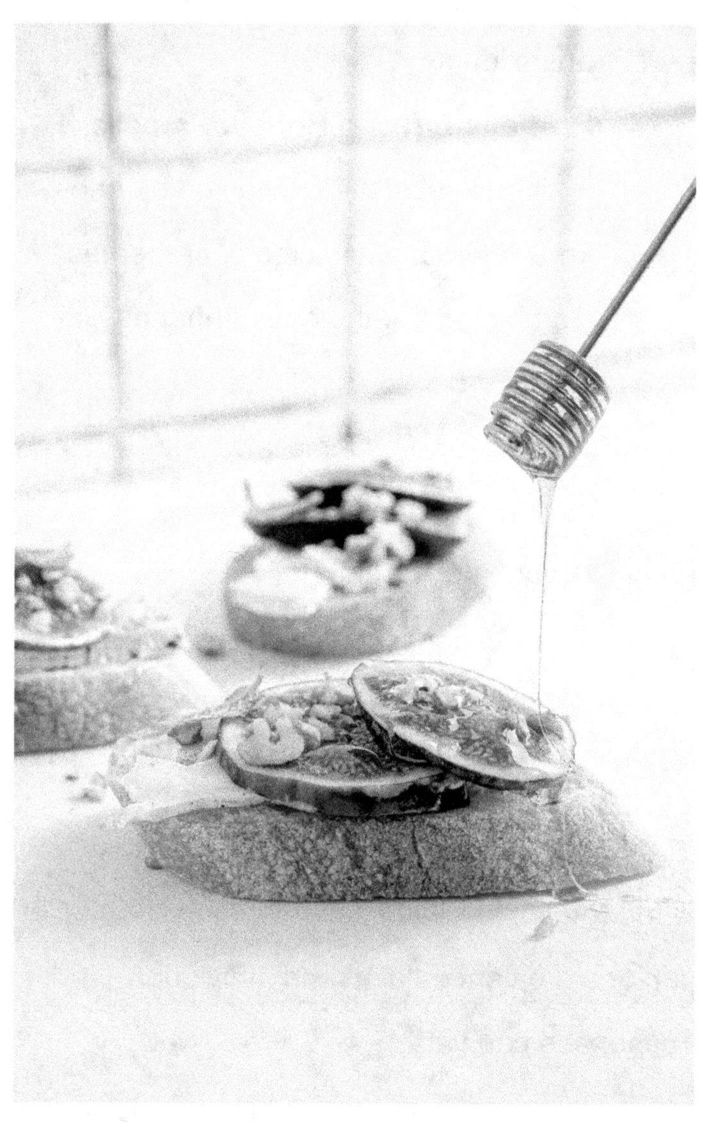

Chapter six

Honey and Cinnamon power

Honey and cinnamon, when combined, create a flavorful and potentially beneficial blend. Some potential health benefits associated with this combination include:

1. **Antioxidant Properties:** Both honey and cinnamon contain antioxidants, which may help neutralize harmful free radicals in the body, supporting overall health.

2. **Anti-Inflammatory Effects:** Cinnamon is known for its anti-inflammatory properties, and honey, especially raw honey, also has potential anti-inflammatory effects. This

combination may help with inflammatory conditions.

3. **Blood Sugar Management:** Some studies suggest that cinnamon may help improve insulin sensitivity and regulate blood sugar levels. When combined with honey, it can create a sweet alternative with potential benefits for those managing diabetes.

4. **Digestive Health:** The mixture of honey and cinnamon may aid in digestion. Honey has natural enzymes, while cinnamon may help alleviate digestive discomfort.

5. **Immune System Support:** Both honey and cinnamon are believed to have immune-boosting properties, which can contribute to overall well-being.

It's important to remember that although these possible advantages could exist, each person's reaction is unique. This combination should be consumed in moderation as part of a balanced diet.

Sweet Stuff: Honey Combos

Honey pairs well with various sweet ingredients, creating delightful combinations. Here are some sweet stuff honey combos:

1. **Honey and Nut Butter:** Spread honey on toast or drizzle it over nut butter (such as almond or peanut butter) for a delicious and nutritious treat.
2. **Yogurt and Honey:** Mix honey into yogurt for a naturally sweet and creamy

snack. Add some fruits or nuts for extra flavor and texture.

3. **Fruits and Honey:** Drizzle honey over fresh fruits like berries, apples, or melons to enhance their natural sweetness.

4. **Cheese and Honey:** Pair honey with cheese, such as brie or goat cheese, for a delightful balance of sweetness and savory richness.

5. **Oatmeal and Honey:** Stir honey into your morning oatmeal or granola for a sweet and satisfying breakfast.

6. **Tea and Honey:** Sweeten your tea with honey instead of sugar for a soothing and natural flavor enhancer.

7. **Desserts and Honey:** Use honey as a sweetener in baking or drizzle it over desserts like ice cream, pancakes, or

waffles for an added touch of sweetness.

Experimenting with these combinations allows you to enjoy the versatility of honey in various sweet treats.

Tea and Honey

Tea and honey form a classic pairing that goes beyond simple sweetness. Here are some aspects of this combination:

1. **Natural Sweetener:** Honey serves as a natural sweetener for tea, offering a pleasant sweetness without the refined sugars found in many sweeteners.
2. **Flavor Enhancement:** Honey adds depth and complexity to the flavor profile of tea. Different honey varieties, such as

clover or orange blossom, can impart
unique notes to your brew.

3. **Antioxidant Boost:** Both tea and honey
   contain antioxidants that may contribute
   to overall health. Combining them
   provides a tasty way to enjoy these
   potential benefits.

4. **Soothing Qualities:** The warmth of tea,
   combined with the soothing properties of
   honey, can provide comfort, making it a
   popular choice for those seeking a
   calming and enjoyable beverage.

5. **Variety of Combinations:** Experiment
   with different teas, such as black, green,
   or herbal, paired with various honey
   varieties to discover your preferred
   flavor combinations.

Whether you're sipping a hot cup of tea on a chilly day or enjoying a refreshing iced tea, the addition of honey enhances the experience, making it a timeless and versatile pairing.

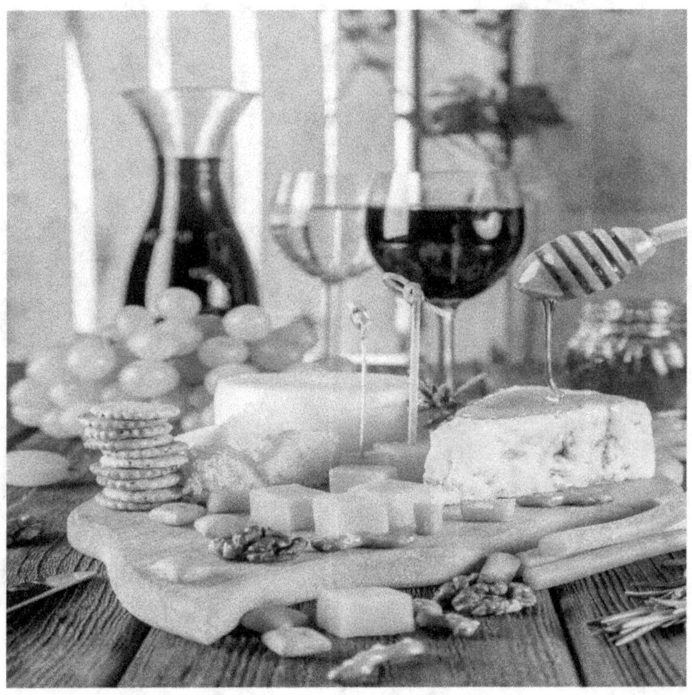

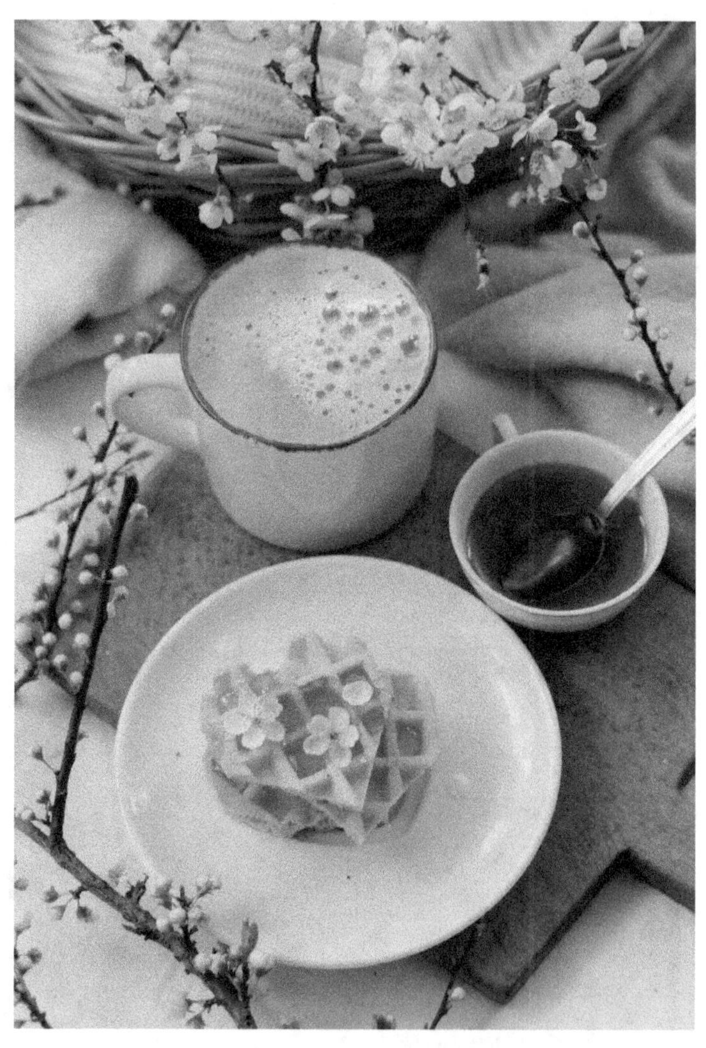

Chapter seven

Home Cures

While I can provide general information, it's crucial to note that home remedies or "cures" should not replace professional medical advice. However, here are some common home remedies that people find helpful for certain situations:

1. **Honey and Lemon for Sore Throat:** Mix honey with warm water and a squeeze of lemon to soothe a sore throat. Honey's antibacterial properties may offer relief.

2. **Ginger Tea for Nausea:** Ginger tea can be soothing for nausea. You can make it

by steeping fresh ginger slices in hot water or using ginger tea bags.

3. **Saltwater Gargle for Sore Throat:** Gargling with warm saltwater can help alleviate a sore throat by reducing inflammation and killing bacteria.

4. **Peppermint Oil for Headaches:** Applying diluted peppermint oil to your temples may provide relief from tension headaches. Be cautious with essential oils and use them as directed.

5. **Chamomile Tea for Sleep:** Chamomile tea is known for its calming properties and may help promote relaxation and improve sleep quality.

6. **Aloe Vera for Sunburn:** Apply aloe vera gel to sunburned skin for its soothing and cooling effects.

7. **Turmeric and Honey for Wounds:** A
   mixture of turmeric and honey can
   create a paste with potential
   antibacterial properties that may aid in
   wound healing.

Always consult with a healthcare professional before trying home remedies, especially if you have underlying health conditions or if symptoms persist. Home remedies are not a substitute for proper medical care when needed.

Home remedies for your Kitchen

Certainly, many common kitchen ingredients can serve as home remedies for various purposes. Here are a few examples:

1. **Baking Soda:**

   - For Heartburn: Mix a teaspoon of baking soda in a glass of water to help neutralize stomach acid.
   - For Skin Irritations: Create a paste with water and apply it to soothe minor skin irritations.

2. **Apple Cider Vinegar:**

   - For Sore Throat: Gargle with diluted apple cider vinegar to alleviate throat discomfort.
   - For Digestion: Consuming a diluted solution before meals may aid digestion.

3. **Oatmeal:**

   - For Skin Irritation: Oatmeal baths can help soothe itchy or irritated skin.

4. **Coconut Oil:**

- For Dry Skin: Apply coconut oil to moisturize and soothe dry skin.
    - For Oil Pulling: Swishing coconut oil in your mouth may promote oral health.

5. **Ginger:**
    - For Nausea: Ginger tea or ginger chews can help alleviate nausea.
    - For Joint Pain: Ginger may have anti-inflammatory properties; consider incorporating it into your diet.

6. **Garlic:**
    - For Immune Support: Garlic is believed to have immune-boosting properties when included in your diet.

7. **Honey:**

- For Cough: A teaspoon of honey can be soothing for a cough. Mix it with warm water or tea.

Always be mindful of allergies and consult with a healthcare professional if you have specific health concerns. While these kitchen remedies can offer relief for minor issues, they are not substitutes for professional medical advice and treatment.

Chapter eight

Honey for household

Honey isn't just a sweetener; it has various household uses. Here are some ways you can incorporate honey into your household:

1. **Natural Sweetener:**
   - Use honey as a healthier alternative to refined sugar in cooking and baking.
2. **Soothing Cough Remedy:**
   - Mix honey with warm water or tea to soothe a sore throat or alleviate coughing.
3. **Facial Mask:**
   - Create a natural facial mask by combining honey with ingredients

like yogurt or oats. It may aid in skin calming and moisturization.

4. **Homemade Salad Dressing:**
   - Use honey to sweeten and balance flavors in homemade salad dressings.

5. **Preserving Fruits:**
   - Coat cut fruits like apples with honey to slow down browning.

6. **Natural Energy Boost:**
   - Consume a spoonful of honey for a quick and natural energy boost.

7. **Wound Healing:**
   - Apply honey to minor cuts or burns; its antibacterial properties may aid in the healing process.

8. **Hair Conditioner:**

o   Make a hair mask by mixing
    honey with olive oil to condition
    and add shine to your hair.

9. **Wood Polish:**

    o   Mix equal parts of olive oil and
        honey to create a natural wood
        polish for furniture.

10. **Candle Holder Cleaner:**

    o   Use a mixture of honey and water
        to clean and polish candle
        holders.

Ensure you are using pure honey for these applications, and remember that while honey has beneficial properties, it's essential to seek professional advice for specific health concerns or conditions.

The joy of cooking with honey

Cooking with honey adds a natural sweetness and depth to dishes. It can be a versatile ingredient in both sweet and savory recipes, enhancing flavors and providing a unique touch. From glazes for meats to drizzling on desserts, honey brings a delightful richness to your culinary creations.

Honey recipes

Certainly! Here are a few diverse honey-infused recipes to try:

1. **Honey Garlic Chicken:**
   - Combine honey, soy sauce, minced garlic, and ginger.

Marinate chicken, then bake or grill for a flavorful dish.

2. **Honey Mustard Salad Dressing:**

    o   Mix honey, Dijon mustard, olive oil, and a splash of apple cider vinegar for a sweet and tangy salad dressing.

3. **Honey Lemon Ginger Tea:**

    o   Brew a cup of hot tea, add honey for sweetness, and a slice of fresh ginger with a squeeze of lemon for a soothing beverage.

4. **Spicy Honey Glazed Shrimp:**

    o   Toss shrimp in a glaze made of honey, chili flakes, soy sauce, and a touch of lime juice. Cook until glazed and serve over rice or salad.

5. **Honey Yogurt Parfait:**

- Layer Greek yogurt with honey, granola, and fresh berries for a delicious and healthy parfait.

6. **Honey Sesame Stir-Fry:**

   - Stir-fry your favorite veggies and protein in a sauce made with honey, soy sauce, garlic, and sesame oil.

7. **Honey Nut Granola Bars:**

   - Mix oats, nuts, dried fruits, and honey. Press into a pan and bake for homemade granola bars.

8. **Honey Balsamic Roasted Vegetables:**

   - Toss your choice of vegetables in a mixture of honey, balsamic vinegar, olive oil, and roast until caramelized.

9. **Honey Lemon Glazed Salmon:**

- Combine honey, lemon juice, and soy sauce as a glaze for baked or grilled salmon.

10. **Honey Cinnamon Butter:**
    - Mix honey, softened butter, and a dash of cinnamon. Spread on toast, muffins, or pancakes.

Remember to adjust quantities according to your taste preferences, and feel free to get creative with these honey-inspired recipes!

Honey Resources

For honey resources, consider local beekeepers, farmers' markets, or specialty grocery stores. Online platforms like Beekeeping Associations or websites dedicated to raw, organic honey can provide a variety of options. Understanding different types, such as wildflower or clover honey, enhances your culinary experience. Always prioritize quality and authenticity when exploring honey resources.

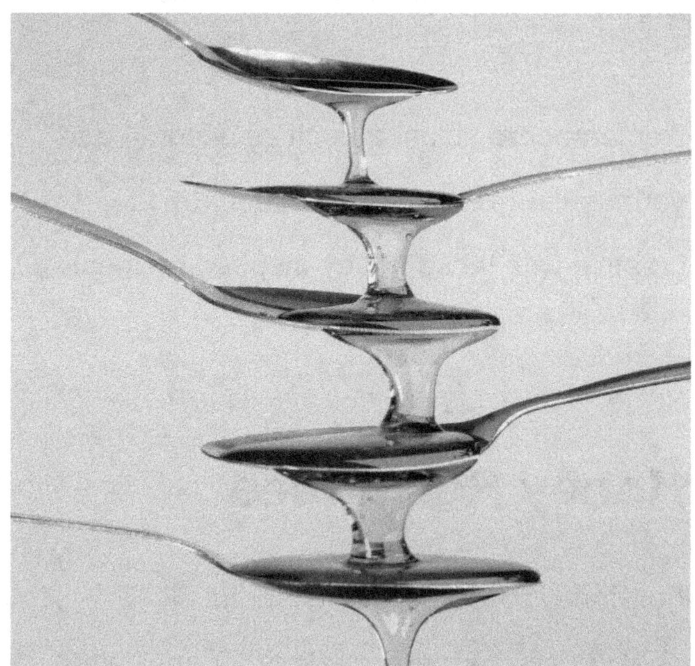

Conclusion

In conclusion, the myriad health benefits attributed to honey underscore its remarkable healing powers. From its potent antimicrobial properties to its soothing effects on respiratory issues, honey has proven to be a versatile and natural remedy. Its rich history in traditional medicine and the scientific evidence supporting its therapeutic qualities make honey a valuable addition to holistic healthcare practices. Embracing the healing powers of honey not only taps into centuries-old wisdom but also aligns with contemporary efforts to explore nature's remedies for a healthier lifestyle.

www.ingramcontent.com/pod-product-compliance
Lightning Source LLC
Chambersburg PA
CBHW071120260726
48661CB00006B/2654

9 798876 538543